Effortless Cooking

30 Easy & Delicious Pureed Recipe Fit for all Ages

By

Jennifer Jones

© 2019 Jennifer Jones, All Rights Reserved.

License Notices

The book, hereunto known as "The Book" shall not be copied or reproduced in any way without the express permission of the "The Author". "The Book" is licensed for single use and is not transferable. If you are in possession of an illegal download of "The Book", delete your version and purchase a new one.

The opinions, suggestions, directions and guidelines mentioned in "The Book" are strictly for informational use. The Author has gone to great lengths to ensure authenticity, but accepts no liability for any commercial or personal damage incurred by misinterpretation of "The Book". The Reader assumes all risk when following the content of the "The Book".

Get Your Daily Deals Here!

Thanks for buying my book! As a special offer, you are now eligible for free books when you sign up below. All you need to do is fill in your email address and offers will be emailed to you on a daily basis for free and discounted books. To make sure you never miss one of these unique offers, a reminder email will be sent to you a few days before the offer expires. You don't have to do a thing! Subscribe now in the box below and start receiving your thank you gift!

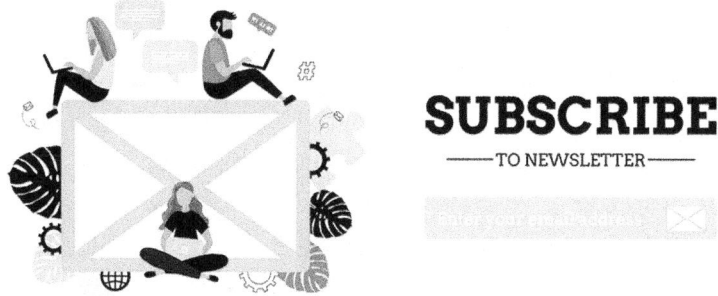

https://Jennifer-Jones.gr8.com

Table of Contents

Easy and Delicious Pureed Recipes 7

    Recipe 1: Avocado Puree 8

    Recipe 2: Peach Puree 10

    Recipe 3: Pureed Sweet Potato 12

    Recipe 4: Apple Puree 14

    Recipe 5: Pureed Carrots 16

    Recipe 6: Banana Puree 18

    Recipe 7: Quinoa and Vegetable soup 20

    Recipe 8: Apple & Banana Puree 22

    Recipe 9: Split Pea & Quinoa Soup 24

    Recipe 10: Mango Puree 26

    Recipe 11: Coconut Mushroom Soup 28

    Recipe 12: Banana & Mango Puree 30

    Recipe 13: Chestnut Soup 32

Recipe 14: Quinoa, Banana, Apple & Date Puree 35

Recipe 15: Cream of Corn Soup 37

Recipe 16: Nectarine Puree 40

Recipe 17: Creamy Cauliflower Soup 42

Recipe 18: Plum Puree 45

Recipe 19: Butternut Squash, Curried Carrot, and Sweet Potato Soup 47

Recipe 20: Kiwi Puree 50

Recipe 21: Spring Onion and Peas Soup 52

Recipe 22: Chikoo Puree 55

Recipe 23: Summer Berry Puree 57

Recipe 24: Papaya Puree 59

Recipe 25: Tropical Fruit Puree 61

Recipe 26: Guava Puree 63

Recipe 27: Blueberry Puree 65

Recipe 28: Date Puree 67

Recipe 29: Avocado & Banana Puree 69

Recipe 30: Apple and Raspberry Puree 71

About the Author 73

Author's Afterthoughts 75

Easy and Delicious Pureed Recipes

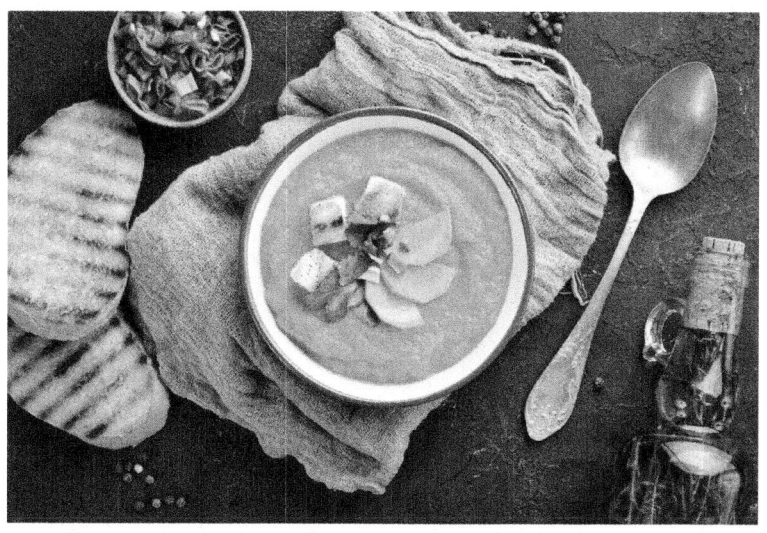

Recipe 1: Avocado Puree

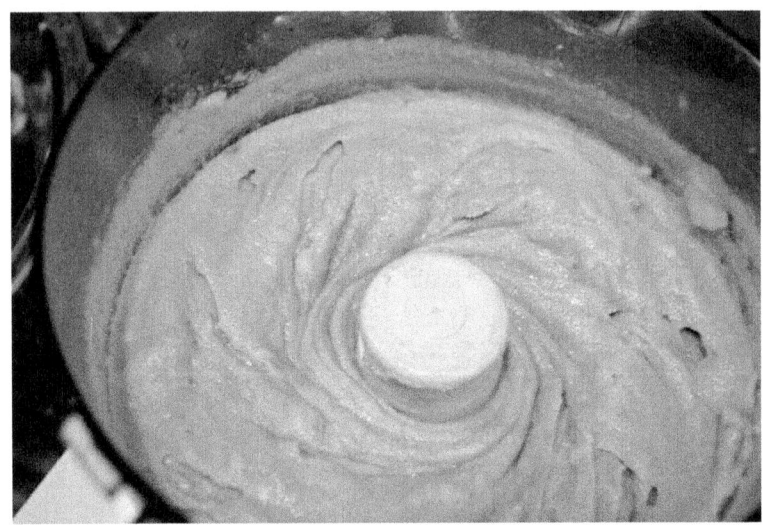

This puree is made from healthy fat and is perfect for babies as is or for adults served alongside dinner and breakfast sandwiches.

Yield: 2

Preparation Time: 15 minutes

Ingredient List:

- Avocado (1, ripe, peeled, seeded and chopped)

HHHHHHHHHHHHHHHHHHHHHHHHHHHHHHHHHHHH

Instructions:

1. Add your avocado pieces with water into a blender or food processor.

2. Serve, and enjoy!

Recipe 2: Peach Puree

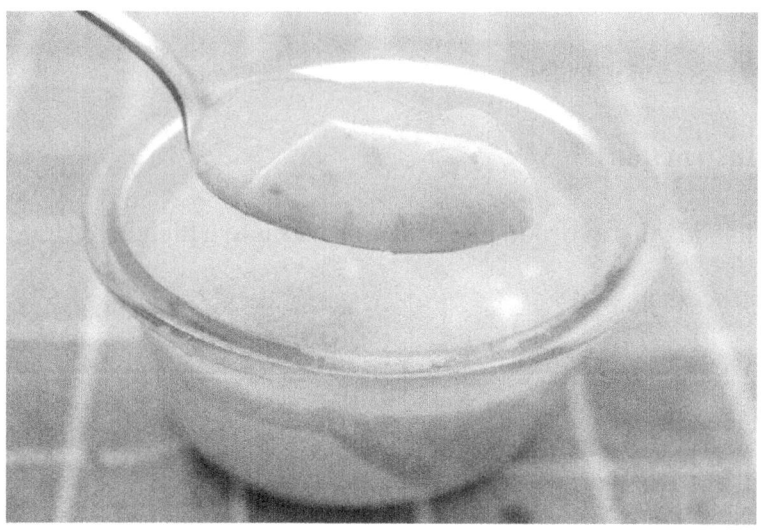

This puree provides a delicious way to add some potassium and beta-carotene to your diet.

Yield: 1 – 2

Preparation Time: 15 minutes

Ingredient List:

- Peaches (2, ripe, peeled, seeded, chopped)
- Water (1 cup)
- Vinegar (1/3 cup)

НННННННННННННННННННННННННННННННННННННН

Instructions:

1. Wash your peach pieces in a water and vinegar mixture.

2. Rinse under cool water then add a cup of water to a pot and bring to a boil.

3. Add in peaches cover and leave for about 45 seconds.

4. Remove from heat and transfer immediately into a container with ice.

5. Transfer your peaches to a blender or food processor until smooth.

6. Serve and enjoy.

Recipe 3: Pureed Sweet Potato

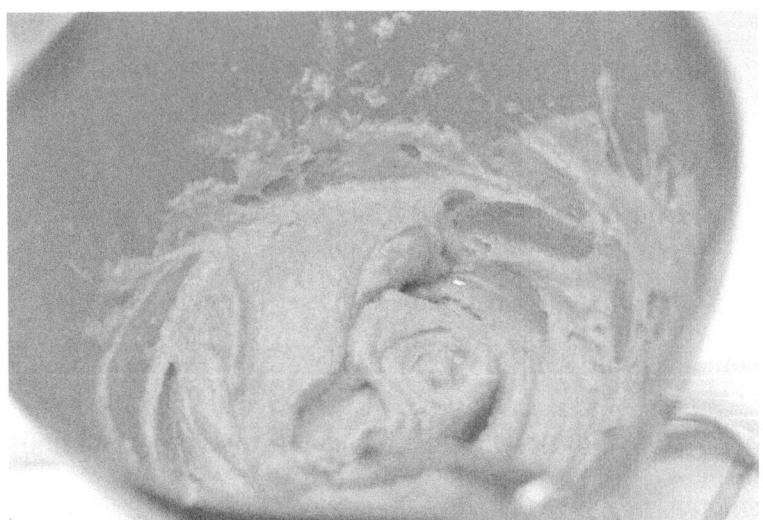

This recipe is a perfect snack or side dish for any age group.

Yield: 4

Preparation Time: 35 minutes

Ingredient List:

- Sweet potato (2lbs., peeled, chopped)
- Salt (1 teaspoon)
- Pepper (1 teaspoon ground)

HHHHHHHHHHHHHHHHHHHHHHHHHHHHHHHHHHHH

Instructions:

5. Set your sweet potato on in a thick bottom pan with just enough water to cover your potato pieces.

6. Cover, and allow to cook until fork tender (about 20 minutes).

7. Strain then add your sweet potato to a food processor or blender and process until smooth.

8. Serve and enjoy.

Recipe 4: Apple Puree

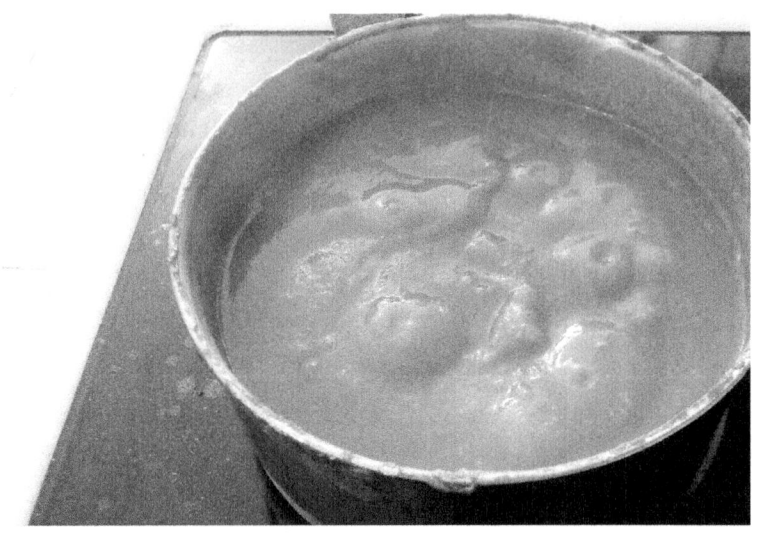

This recipe is perfect for babies.

Yield: 2

Preparation Time: 30 minutes

Ingredient List:

- Apple (1, peeled, cored and chopped)
- Cinnamon (¼ teaspoons)
- Milk (1/8 cup)

HHHHHHHHHHHHHHHHHHHHHHHHHHHHHHHHHHHH

Instructions:

1. Set your apples on in a thick bottom pan with just enough water to cover your apple pieces.

2. Cover, and allow to cook until fork tender (about 7 minutes).

3. Strain then add your apples to a food processor or blender with milk and process until smooth.

4. Transfer to a serving bowl, top with cinnamon and serve.

Recipe 5: Pureed Carrots

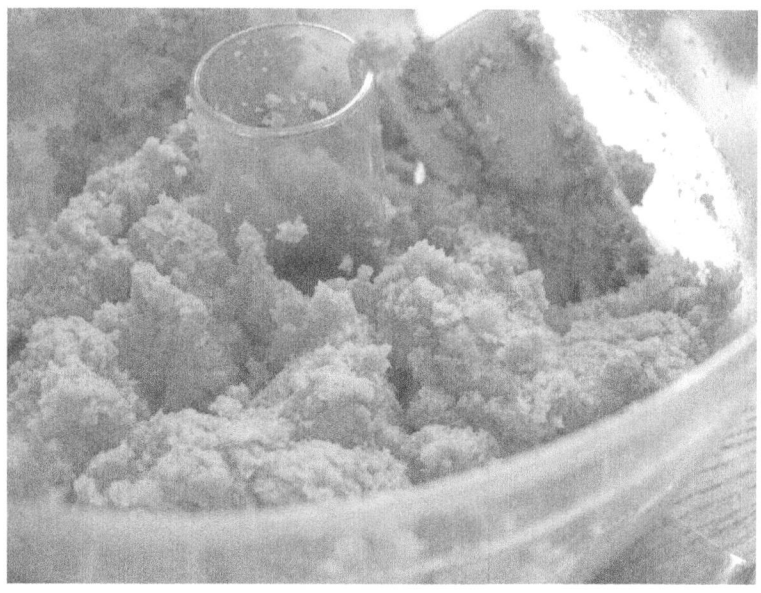

This pureed carrot recipe can serve as a delicious side dish for adults or a full meal for babies.

Yield: 4

Preparation Time: 35 minutes

Ingredient List:

- Carrots (2lbs., peeled, chopped)
- Salt (1 teaspoon)
- Pepper (1 teaspoon ground)

HHHHHHHHHHHHHHHHHHHHHHHHHHHHHHHHHHHH

Instructions:

1. Set your carrots on in a thick bottom pan with just enough water to cover your carrot pieces.

2. Cover, and allow to cook until fork tender (about 20 minutes).

3. Strain then add your carrots to a food processor or blender and process until smooth.

4. Serve and enjoy.

Recipe 6: Banana Puree

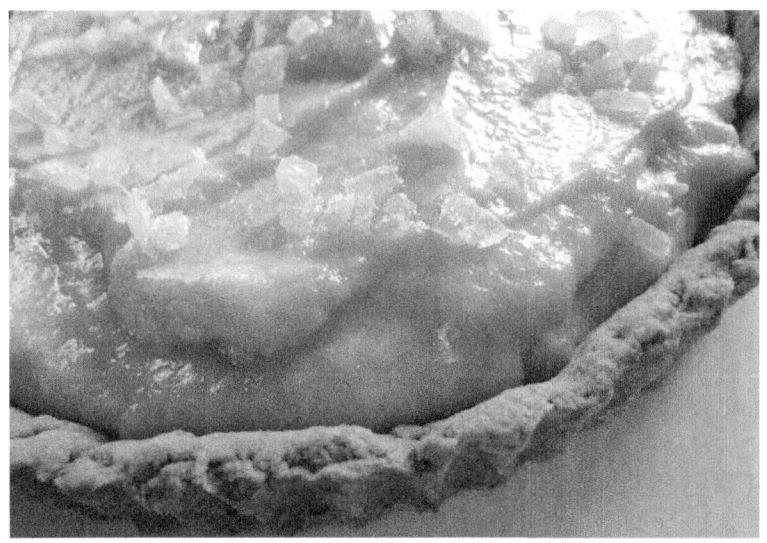

This puree is a perfect snack for babies as early as 4 months old, and adults alike.

Yield: 1

Preparation Time: 15 minutes

Ingredient List:

- Banana (1, ripe, peeled and cut)
- Water (1 tablespoon)

HHHHHHHHHHHHHHHHHHHHHHHHHHHHHHHHHHHH

Instructions:

1. Add banana pieces into a blender or food processor with water and process until smooth.

2. Serve and enjoy.

Recipe 7: Quinoa and Vegetable soup

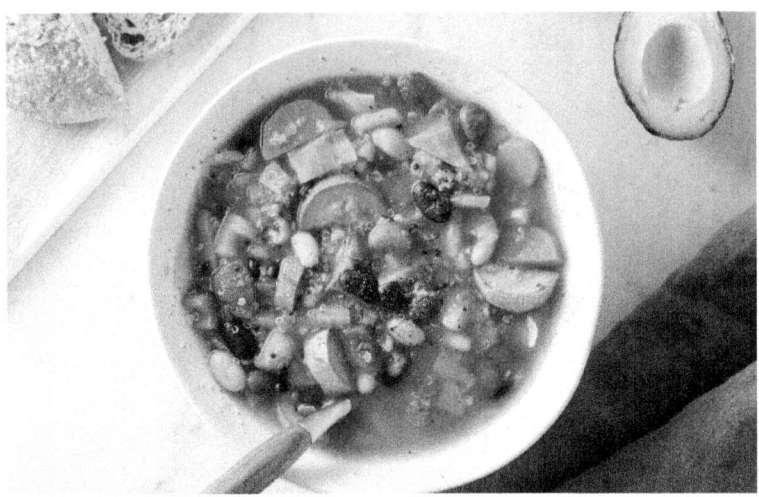

This healthy soup is a combination of quinoa, celery, and smoky flavor coming from the fire roasted tomatoes.

Yield: 8

Preparation Time: 50 minutes

Ingredient List:

- 8oz. can fire roasted tomatoes
- 2 carrots, diced
- 6 cups vegetable broth
- ¼ teaspoon ground coriander seeds
- 1 tablespoon olive oil
- 8oz. Quinoa uncooked
- 2 celery stalks, chopped
- ¼ teaspoon ground cumin
- Salt and pepper, to taste

HHHHHHHHHHHHHHHHHHHHHHHHHHHHHHHH

Instructions:

1. Place all ingredients in a cooker.

2. Stir and set the cooker to simmer.

3. Cook for 45 minutes. Season to taste before serving.

Recipe 8: Apple & Banana Puree

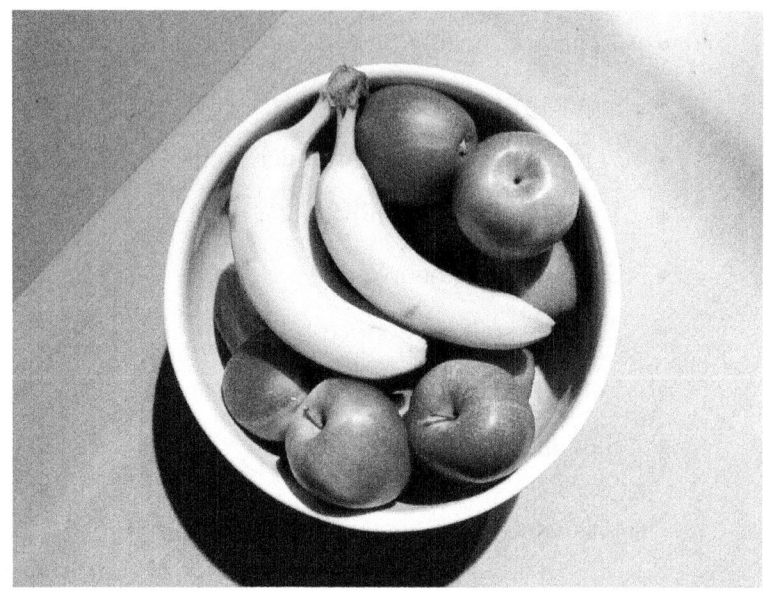

This puree aids in constipation and is perfect for babies and seniors alike.

Yield: 2

Preparation Time: 15 minutes

Ingredient List:

- Apples (2, peeled, cored, and chopped)
- Banana (1, peeled, chopped)

HHHHHHHHHHHHHHHHHHHHHHHHHHHHHHHHHH

Instructions:

1. Set your apples, and bananas on in a thick bottom pan with just enough water to cover your apple pieces.

2. Cover, and allow to cook until fork tender (about 7 minutes).

3. Strain then add your apple and banana to a food processor or blender and process until smooth.

4. Serve and enjoy.

Recipe 9: Split Pea & Quinoa Soup

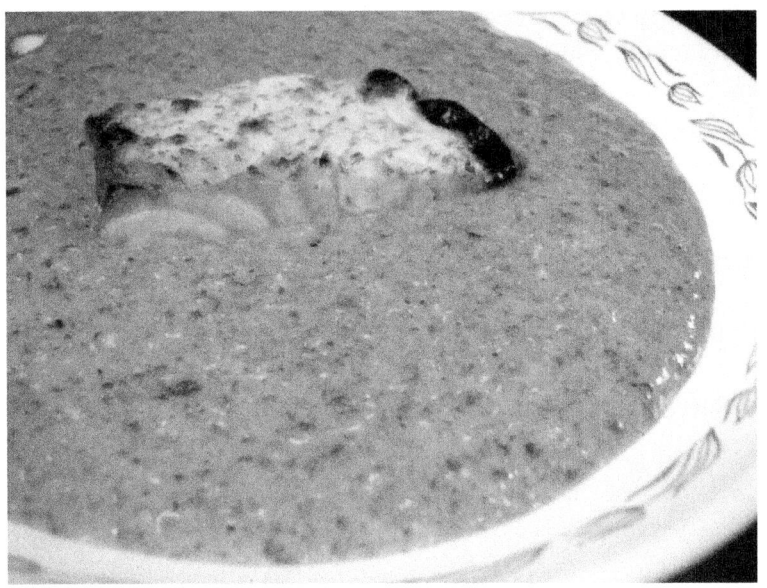

There is nothing better than a hearty soup to end the day.

Yield: 4

Preparation Time: 1 hour

Ingredient List:

- 1 cup yellow split peas
- ½ cup uncooked Quinoa
- 4 cups vegetable broth
- ½ bay leaf
- ¼ teaspoon ground coriander seeds
- ½ tablespoon olive oil
- Salt and pepper, to taste

HHHHHHHHHHHHHHHHHHHHHHHHHHHHHHHH

Instructions:

1. Rinse the peas under cold water and remove any black ones.

2. Place the rinsed peas into a saucepan.

3. Add the remaining ingredients and give it a good stir.

4. Cover and cook for 60 minutes. Season to taste and serve while still hot.

Recipe 10: Mango Puree

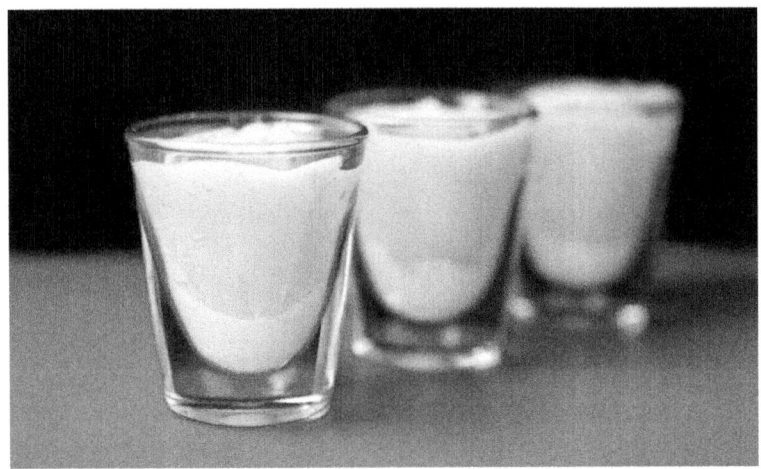

This puree can be given to babies from six months old and older less than 3 days each week.

Yield: 1

Preparation Time: 15 minutes

Ingredient List:

- Mango (1, ripe, peeled, seeded, and chopped)
- Water (1 tablespoon)

HHHHHHHHHHHHHHHHHHHHHHHHHHHHHHHHHHH

Instructions:

1. Add your mango pieces with water into a blender or food processor.

2. Serve, and enjoy!

Recipe 11: Coconut Mushroom Soup

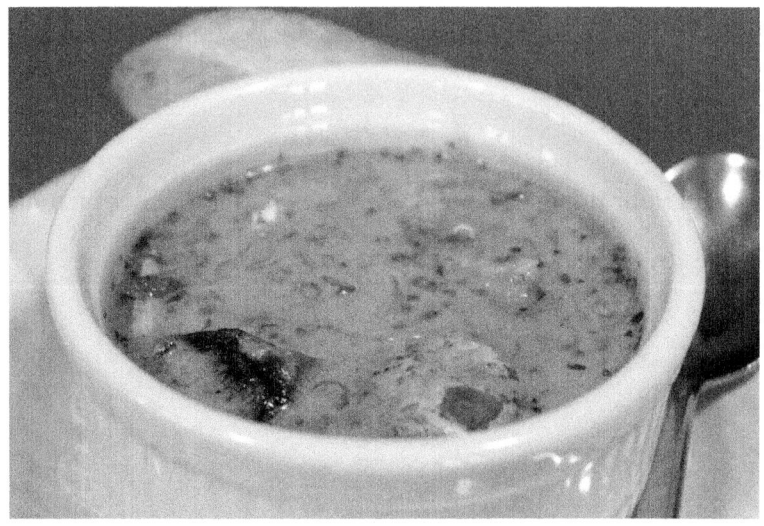

This soup is made with mushrooms cooked in coconut milk.

Yield: 3

Preparation Time: 25 minutes

Ingredient List:

- 1 cup mushrooms, sliced
- 1 cup coconut milk
- 1 onion, sliced
- 1 cup chicken broth
- 4-5 garlic cloves, minced
- ½ teaspoon black pepper
- ¼ teaspoon salt
- 1 tablespoon oil

HHHHHHHHHHHHHHHHHHHHHHHHHHHHHHHHHHH

Instructions:

1. Heat oil in a saucepan, add onion and garlic cloves, cook for 1 minute.

2. Add all mushroom and fry for 5 minutes.

3. Add chicken broth, coconut milk, salt, pepper and mix well.

4. Leave to cook on low heat for 15 minutes.

5. Transfer to serving bowls.

6. Serve and enjoy.

Recipe 12: Banana & Mango Puree

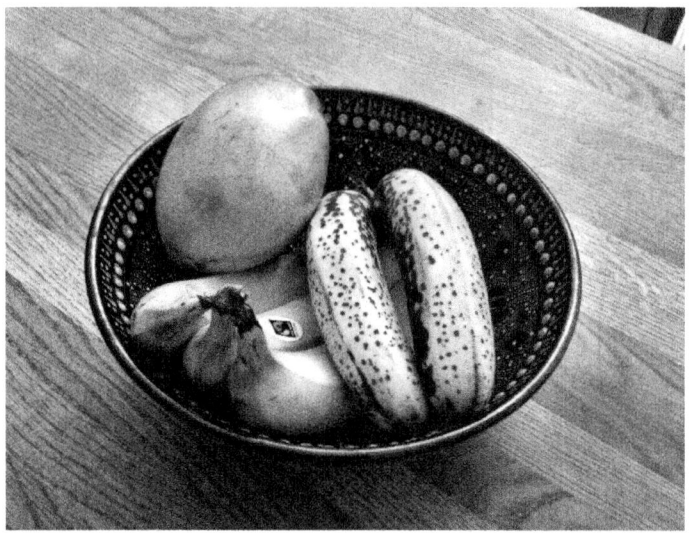

Here is a tropical puree that is delicious for all ages.

Yield: 1

Preparation Time: 15 minutes

Ingredient List:

- Banana (1, ripe, peeled and chopped)
- Mango (1, peeled, seeded and chopped)

Instructions:

1. Add your banana, and mango pieces with water into a blender or food processor.

2. Serve, and enjoy!

Recipe 13: Chestnut Soup

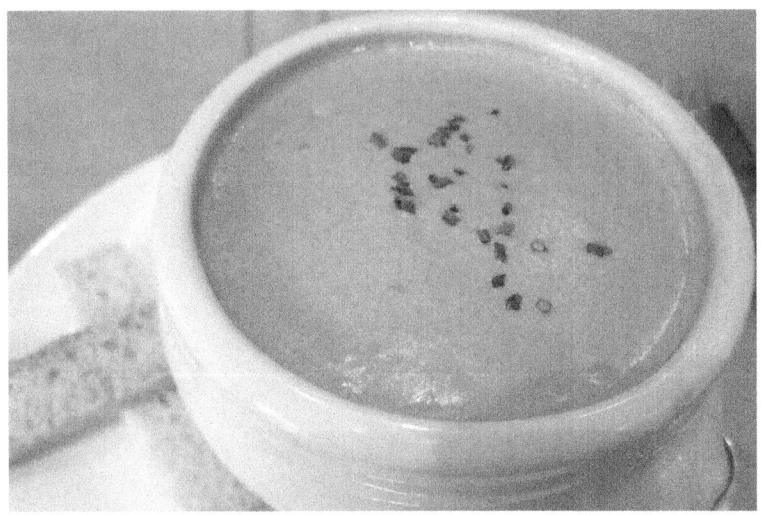

The soup is a combination of heavy cream, roasted chestnuts, and bacon. The perfect soup for the perfect autumn day.

Yield: 6

Preparation Time: 45 minutes

Ingredient List:

- 30oz. whole roasted chestnuts
- 1 shallot, roughly chopped
- bacon slices, chopped
- ½ cup heavy cream
- ½ cups chicken stock
- 1 leek, white and light green parts chopped
- 2 tablespoons butter
- 1 sprig thyme
- 1 bay leaf
- 1 celery stalk, chopped
- ½ teaspoon nutmeg
- Salt and pepper, to taste

HHHHHHHHHHHHHHHHHHHHHHHHHHHHHHHHHHHH

Instructions:

1. Cook bacon in an in a medium saucepot for 3-4 minutes.

2. Add butter, carrot, leek, shallot, and celery. Cook for 6-7 minutes or until veggies is tender.

3. Add stock, thyme, bay leaf, chestnuts and bring to boil. Reduce heat and simmer for 25 minutes.

4. Remove from the heat and discard the thyme and bay leaf. Allow to cool slightly and puree using an immersion blender.

5. Reheat the soup and stir in the cream, nutmeg and season to taste. Cook for 5 minutes more. Serve while still hot.

Recipe 14: Quinoa, Banana, Apple & Date Puree

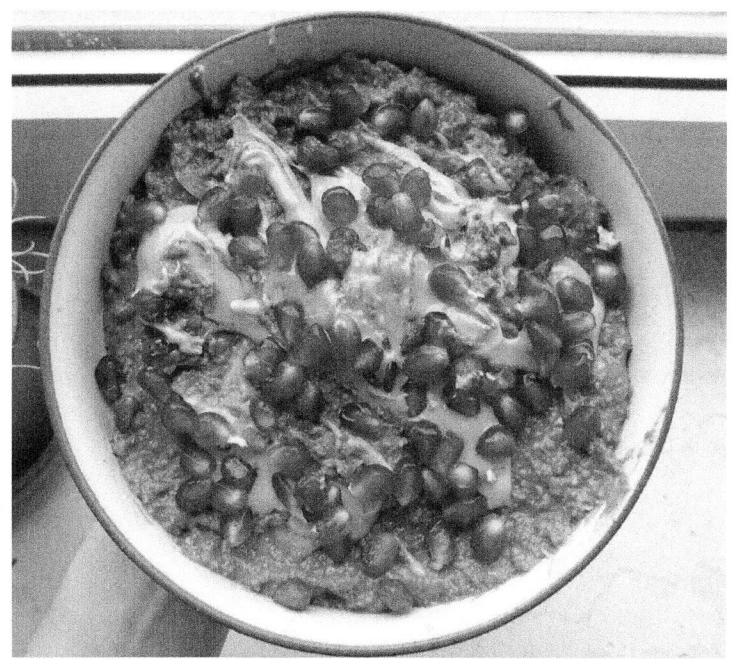

Here is a healthy protein filled puree that is a perfect addition to your baby's diet.

Yield: 1 – 2

Preparation Time: 15 minutes

Ingredient List:

- Quinoa (1 cup, cooked)
- Banana (1, ripe, peeled, chopped)
- Apple (1, ripe, peeled, cored, chopped)
- Dates (6 soft, seeded)
- Cinnamon (¼ teaspoons)

Instructions:

1. Set your apples on in a thick bottom pan with just enough water to cover your apple pieces.

2. Cover, and allow to cook until fork tender (about 7 minutes).

3. Strain then add your apples to a food processor or blender with your quinoa, banana, and dates then process until smooth.

4. Transfer to a serving bowl, top with cinnamon and serve.

Recipe 15: Cream of Corn Soup

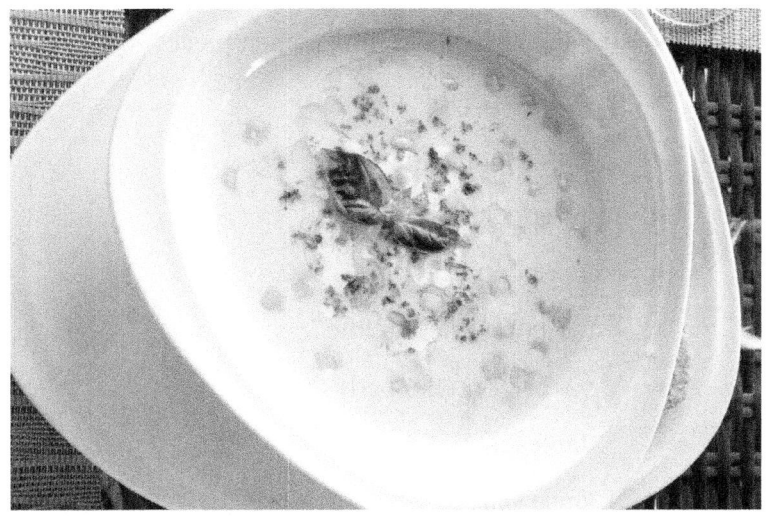

This classic and delicious treat can become even more smooth when finished in a Vitamix.

Yield: 4

Preparation Time: 25 minutes

Ingredient List:

- 0.5 lb. Corn puree
- 0.5 lb. carrots, cut into ½-inch pieces
- 2 cups vegetable stock
- ½ cup chopped onion
- ½ teaspoon Salt
- ¼ teaspoon Pepper
- 1 teaspoon dried thyme
- 2 oz. celery (chopped)
- ½ tablespoon olive oil
- 1 anise star

HHHHHHHHHHHHHHHHHHHHHHHHHHHHHHHHH

Instructions:

1. Heat olive oil in medium pot and add onion; add celery, carrots and sauté for 15 minutes, until onion is caramelized. Add corn and stir until corn is tender.

2. Add thyme and stir well.

3. Transfer the vegetables to a Vitamix, add pumpkin puree, vegetable stock, and pulse until smooth.

4. Transfer the mixture to saucepan and simmer, add anise star and simmer over medium-high heat for 5-8 minutes or until heated through.

5. Remove the anise star and discard.

6. Serve immediately.

Recipe 16: Nectarine Puree

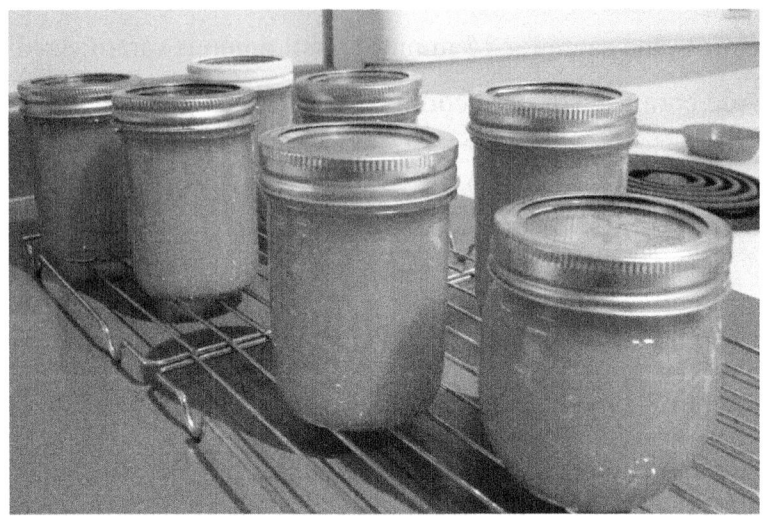

This puree is not only delicious but also provides your body with vitamin C and A.

Yield: 1 – 2

Preparation Time: 15 minutes

Ingredient List:

- Nectarine (2, ripe, peeled, chopped)
- Water (1 cup)
- Vinegar (1/3 cup)

HHHHHHHHHHHHHHHHHHHHHHHHHHHHHHHHHH

Instructions:

1. Wash your nectarine pieces in a water and vinegar mixture.

2. Rinse under cool water then add a cup of water to a pot and bring to a boil.

3. Add in nectarines cover and leave for about 45 seconds.

4. Remove from heat and transfer immediately into a container with ice.

5. Transfer your nectarines to a blender or food processor until smooth.

6. Serve and enjoy.

Recipe 17: Creamy Cauliflower Soup

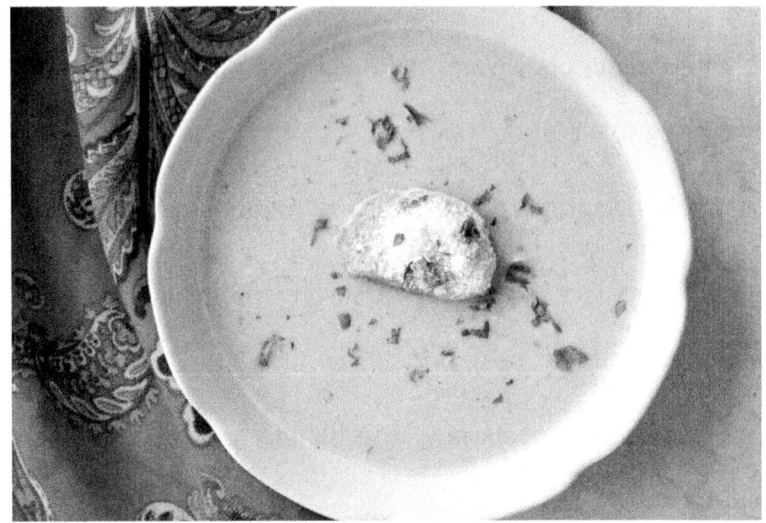

Get a creamy cauliflower soup just like they do in the restaurants.

Yield: 6

Preparation Time: 30 minutes

Ingredient List:

- 14oz. cauliflower heat, cut into florets
- 5oz. watercress
- 7oz. spinach, thawed
- cups chicken stock
- ¼ cup ghee
- Salt and pepper – 1 teaspoon each to taste
- 1 onion, chopped
- 2 garlic cloves, crushed

HHHHHHHHHHHHHHHHHHHHHHHHHHHHHHHHHHHH

Instructions:

1. Grease Dutch oven with ghee, place over the medium-high heat and add onion and garlic. Cook until browned and stir cauliflower florets. Cook for 5 minutes.

2. Add spinach and watercress and cook for 2 minutes or until just wilted, pour in vegetable stock and bring to boil.

3. Cook until cauliflower is crisp-tender and stir in the coconut milk.

4. Season with salt and pepper and remove from the heat. Allow cooling and puree the soup in Vitamix until creamy.

5. Strain and serve immediately.

Recipe 18: Plum Puree

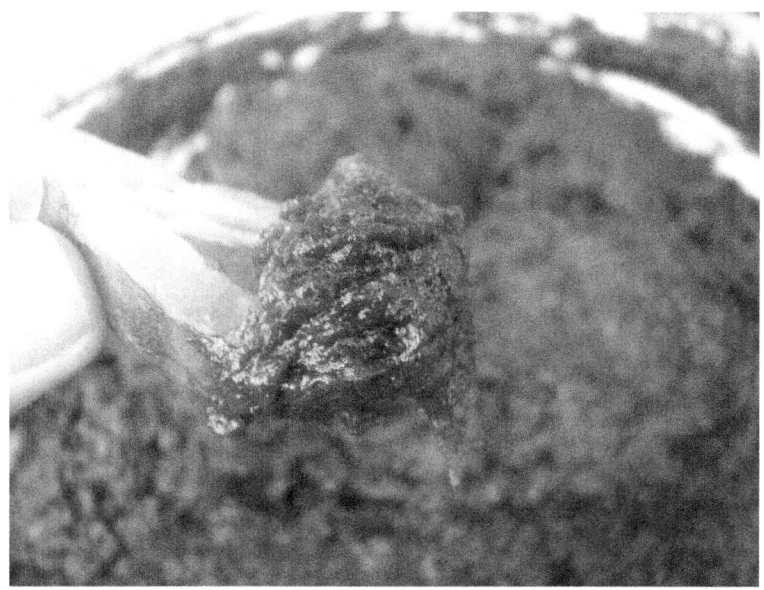

This puree is an amazing source of dietary fiber and is great for constipation.

Yield: 1

Preparation Time: 15 minutes

Ingredient List:

- Plums (6, ripe, pitted)

HHHHHHHHHHHHHHHHHHHHHHHHHHHHHHHHHHHHH

Instructions:

1. Wash your plum pieces in a water and vinegar mixture.

2. Rinse under cool water then add a cup of water to a pot and bring to a boil.

3. Add in plums cover and leave for about 45 seconds.

4. Remove from heat and transfer immediately into a container with ice.

5. Transfer your plums to a blender or food processor until smooth.

6. Serve and enjoy.

Recipe 19: Butternut Squash, Curried Carrot, and Sweet Potato Soup

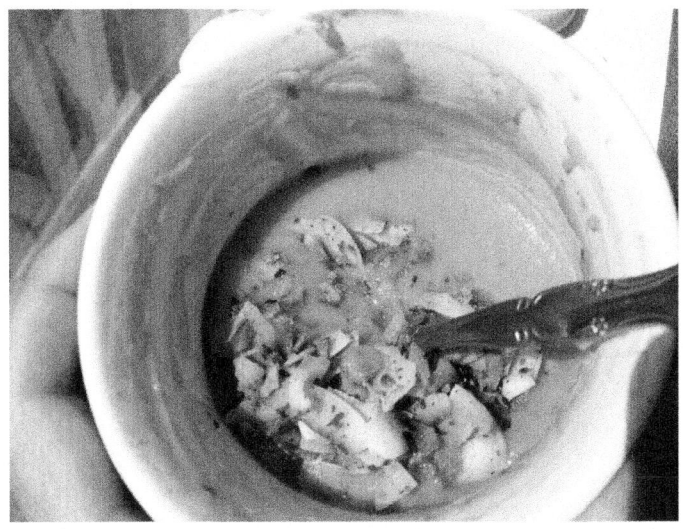

Cholesterol isn't an issue when enjoying this delicious creamy soup, as it Is filled with Beta-Carotene and Vitamin A which together helps to promote healthy vision.

Yield: 3

Preparation Time: 30 – 35min

Ingredient List:

- Extra Virgin Olive Oil (2 teaspoons)
- Shallots (½ cup, chopped)
- Sweet Potato (3 cups, peeled, cubed)
- Carrots (1½ cup, peeled, sliced)
- Butternut Squash (1 cup, peeled, cubed)

HHHHHHHHHHHHHHHHHHHHHHHHHHHHHHHHHHHH

Instructions:

1. Place a saucepan with your oil over medium heat until it just begins to smoke.

2. Add your shallots to the pot and sauté until it becomes tender (should take approximately 2 – 3 min).

3. Add all your prepped vegetables to the shallots, and your curry then allow to cook for another 2 minutes.

4. Pour in your broth and allow it to come to a boil. Once boiling, place the lid on the pot and reduce the heat to low.

5. Allow this mixture to simmer until your vegetables are all tender.

6. Once tender, add salt and pour your soup into a food processor. Pulse until creamy and smooth.

7. Strain, serve and Enjoy.

Tip: Consider topping with a teaspoon of roasted squash seeds.

Recipe 20: Kiwi Puree

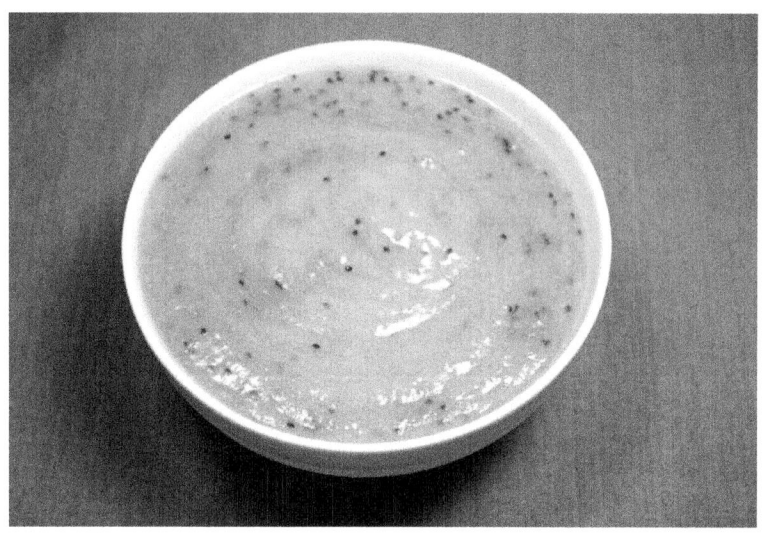

This tropical puree is rich in fiber and vitamins C and A.

Yield: 1

Time Needed: 15 minutes

Ingredient List:

- Kiwi (1, ripe, peeled and chopped)

HHHHHHHHHHHHHHHHHHHHHHHHHHHHHHHHHHHHH

Instructions:

1. Add kiwi pieces into a blender or food processor with water and process until smooth.

2. Serve and enjoy.

Recipe 21: Spring Onion and Peas Soup

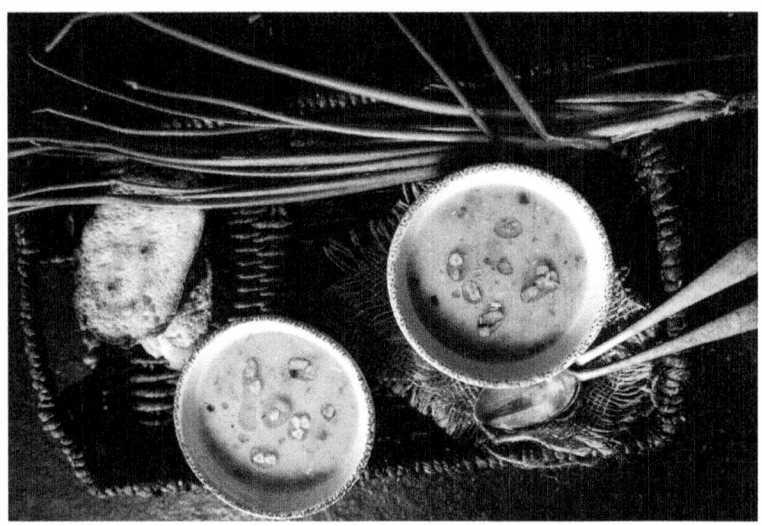

A simple and colorful soup that with blow your mind.

Yield: 3

Preparation Time: 25 minutes

Ingredient List:

- 1 cup peas, boiled
- 2 carrots, peeled, chopped
- 1 bunch spring onion, sliced
- 2 cups chicken broth
- 1 tablespoon lemon juice
- 4-5 garlic cloves, minced
- ½ teaspoon black pepper
- ¼ teaspoon salt
- 1 tablespoon oil

HHHHHHHHHHHHHHHHHHHHHHHHHHHHHHHHHHHH

Instructions:

1. Heat oil in a saucepan, add onion and garlic cloves, fry for 2 minutes.

2. Add all peas and carrots stir for 5 minutes.

3. Add chicken broth, salt, pepper, and mix well.

4. Leave to cook on low heat for 15 minutes.

5. Strain and ladle into serving bowls.

6. Drizzle lemon juice.

7. Serve and enjoy.

Recipe 22: Chikoo Puree

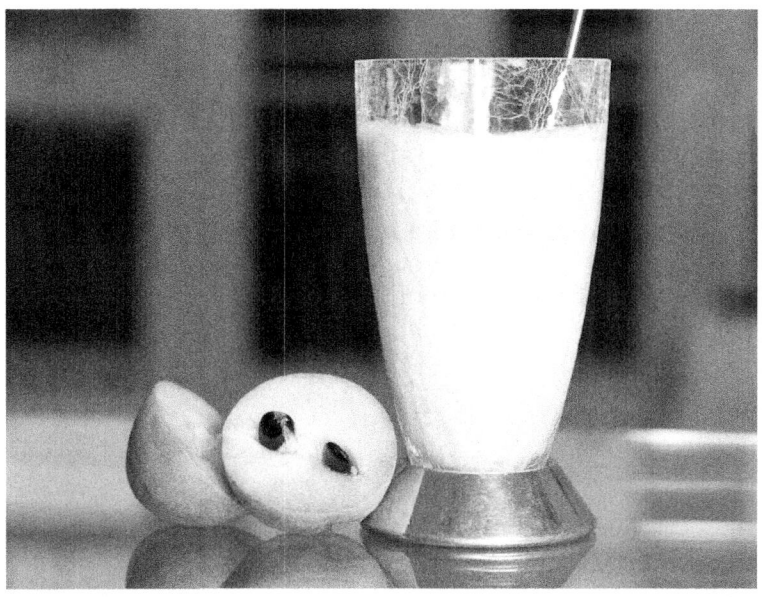

Here is a puree that is great for digestion and maintaining a healthy immune system.

Yield: 1

Preparation Time: 15 minutes

Ingredient List:

- Chikoo (1, ripe, peeled, chopped and seeded)

HHHHHHHHHHHHHHHHHHHHHHHHHHHHHHHHH

Instructions:

1. Add chikoo pieces into a blender or food processor with water and process until smooth.

2. Serve and enjoy.

Recipe 23: Summer Berry Puree

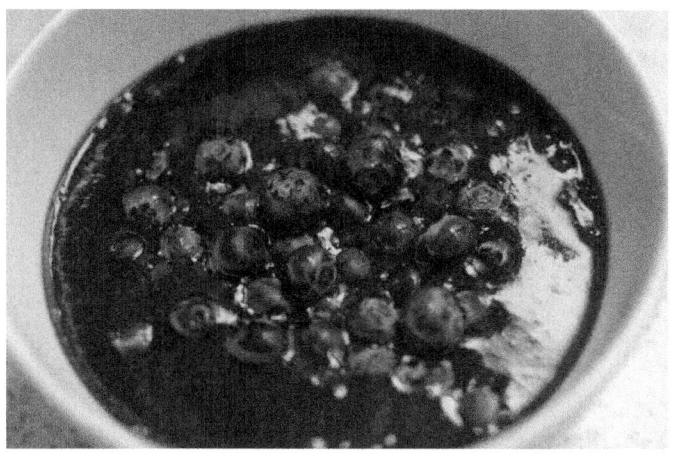

This puree is healthy, tasty, and naturally sweet.

Yield: 3

Preparation Time: 15 minutes

Ingredient List:

- Blueberries (100g)
- Strawberries (100g)
- Raspberries (100g)

HHHHHHHHHHHHHHHHHHHHHHHHHHHHHHHHHHH

Instructions:

1. Wash all your berries and remove any stalks.

2. Add to a blender or food processor then puree until smooth.

3. Strain, serve and enjoy!

Recipe 24: Papaya Puree

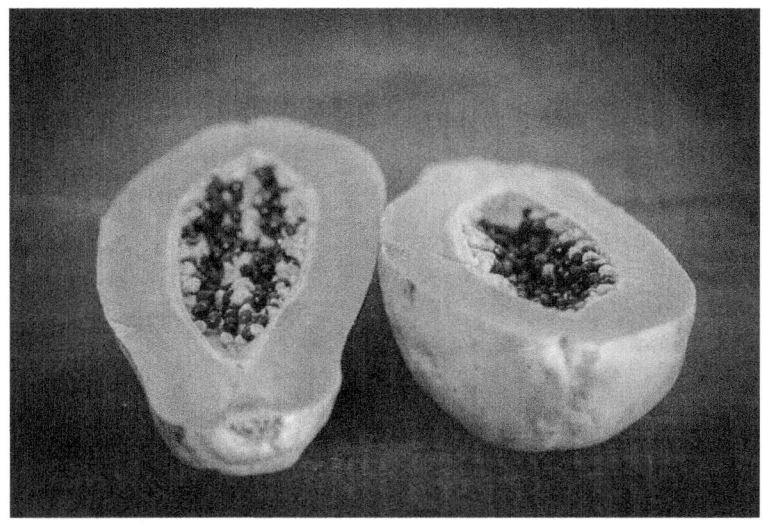

This puree will be a hit with your children due to its natural sweetness.

Yield: 1

Preparation Time: 15 minutes

Ingredient List:

- Papaya (1, ripe, peeled, seeded and chopped)

Instructions:

1. Add papaya pieces into a blender or food processor with water and process until smooth.

2. Serve and enjoy.

Recipe 25: Tropical Fruit Puree

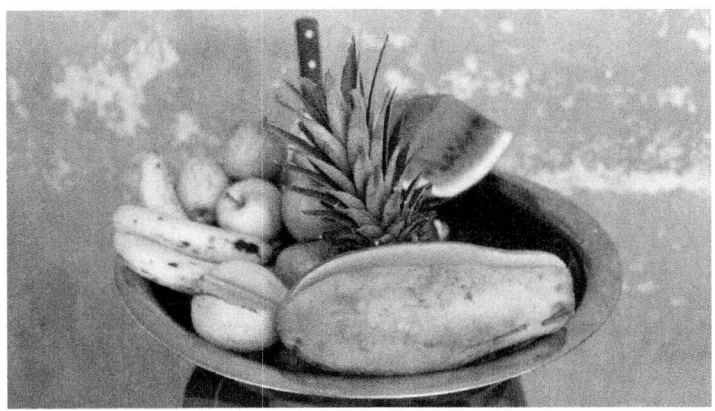

This tropical puree will be a hit with your 6 months or older baby.

Yield: 3 – 4

Preparation Time: 15 minutes

Ingredient List:

- Banana (1, ripe, peeled and chopped)
- Mango (200g, peeled, seeded, chopped)
- Papaya (200g, peeled, seeded, chopped)
- Water (2 tablespoons)

HHHHHHHHHHHHHHHHHHHHHHHHHHHHHHHHHH

Instructions:

1. Add all your chopped fruit to a blender, or food processor then puree until smooth.

2. Serve and enjoy.

Recipe 26: Guava Puree

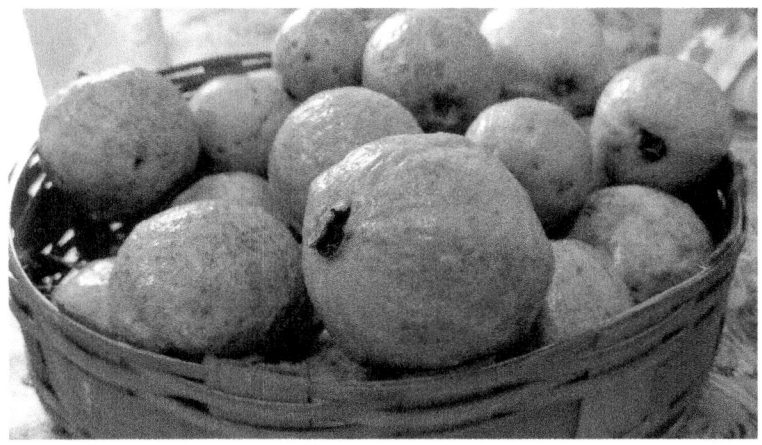

Here is yet another puree that can help you maintain a healthy immune system.

Yield: 1

Preparation Time: 15 minutes

Ingredient List:

- Guava (1, ripe, seeded and chopped)

HHHHHHHHHHHHHHHHHHHHHHHHHHHHHHHHHHH

Instructions:

1. Set your guava on in a thick bottom pan with just enough water to cover your guava pieces.

2. Cover, and allow to cook until fork tender (about 7 minutes).

3. Strain then add your guava to a food processor or blender and process until smooth.

4. Serve and enjoy.

Recipe 27: Blueberry Puree

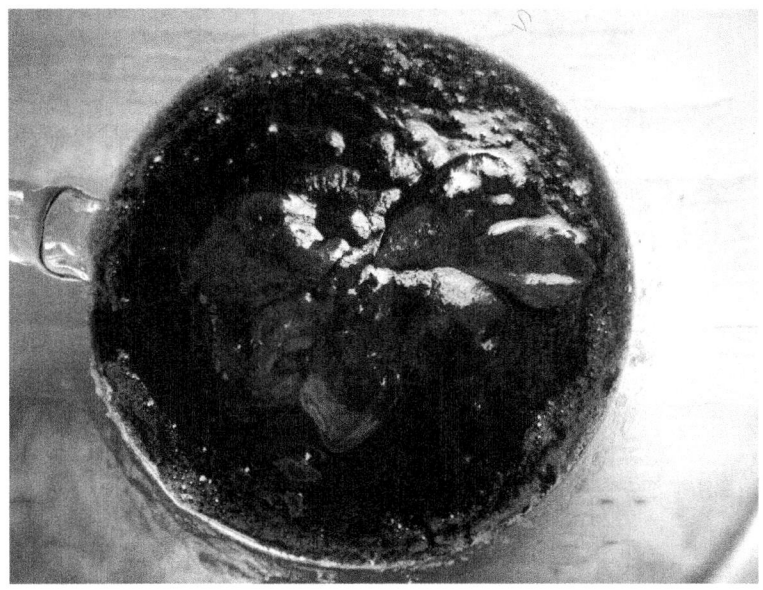

This puree is a delicious and healthy puree that can be served to your children from as early as 8 months.

Yield: 1

Preparation Time: 15 minutes

Ingredient List:

- Blueberries (1 cup)
- Water (½ cup)

HHHHHHHHHHHHHHHHHHHHHHHHHHHHHHHHHHHH

Instructions:

1. Set your berries on in a thick bottom pan with just enough water to cover your apple pieces.

2. Cover, and allow to cook until fork tender (about 7 minutes).

3. Strain then add your berries to a food processor or blender and process until smooth.

4. Serve and enjoy.

Recipe 28: Date Puree

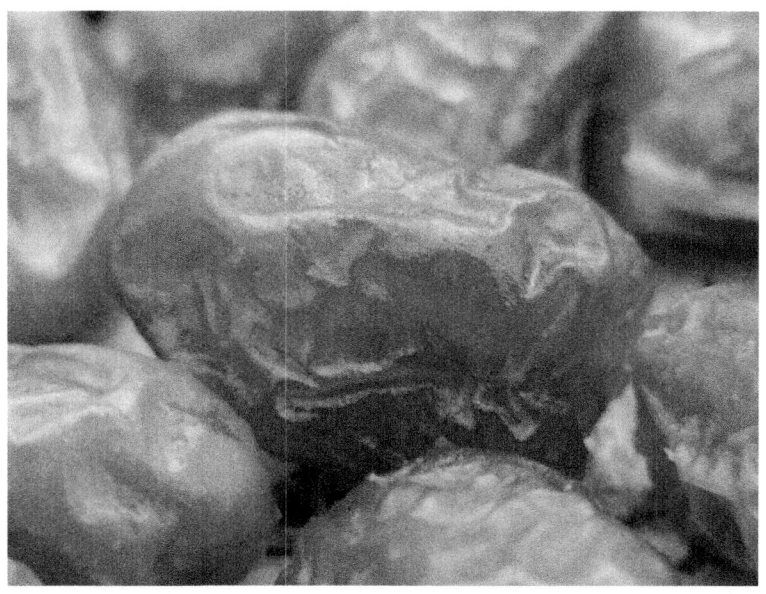

Here is a delicious puree that you can add to your baby's food or your own milkshakes.

Yield: 3

Preparation Time: 15 minutes

Ingredient List:

- Dates (20, seeded)
- Water (1 cup)

HHHHHHHHHHHHHHHHHHHHHHHHHHHHHHHHHHH

Instructions:

1. Add your ingredients in a thick bottom saucepan and allow to cook, boiling for 10 minutes.

2. Cool and transfer the mixture to a blender then puree until smooth.

3. Return the mixture to your saucepan and cook on medium until the puree thickens.

4. Cool, serve, and store the leftovers in an airtight container.

Recipe 29: Avocado & Banana Puree

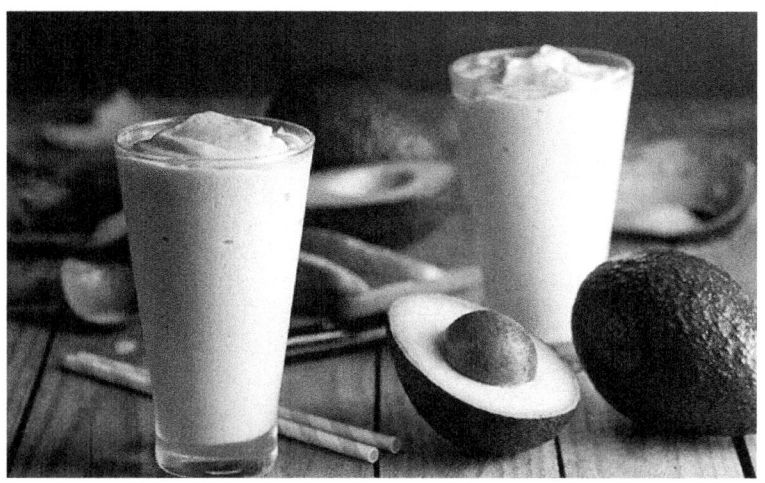

Add healthy fats, and potassium to your diet with this delicious puree.

Yield: 1

Preparation Time: 10 minutes

Ingredient List:

- Banana (½, ripe, peeled, and chopped)
- Avocado (¼, ripe, peeled, and chopped)
- Yoghurt (2 tablespoons)

HHHHHHHHHHHHHHHHHHHHHHHHHHHHHHHHHHHHHHH

Instructions:

1. Add banana, and avocado pieces into a blender or food processor with water and process until smooth.

2. Serve and enjoy.

Recipe 30: Apple and Raspberry Puree

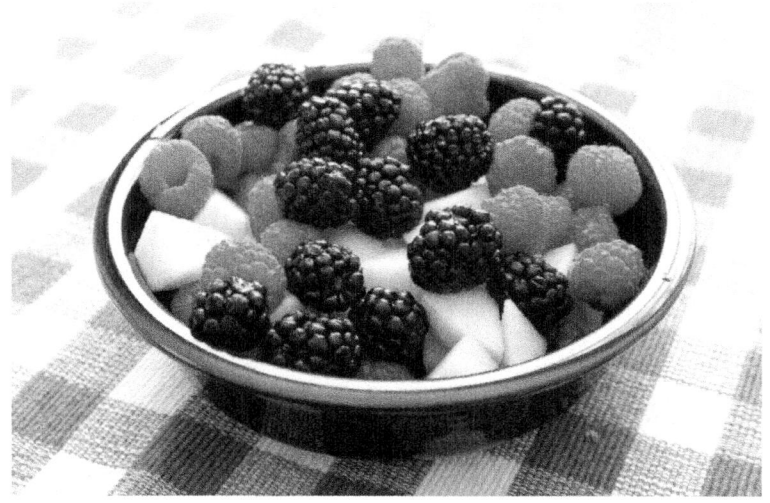

This naturally sweet puree is perfect for the whole family.

Yield: 3

Preparation Time: 15 minutes

Ingredient List:

- Apple (1, ripe, peeled, cored, and chopped)
- Raspberries (100g)

HHHHHHHHHHHHHHHHHHHHHHHHHHHHHHHHHHH

Instructions:

1. Set your apple, and raspberries on in a thick bottom pan with just enough water to cover your apple pieces.

2. Cover, and allow to cook until fork tender (about 7 minutes).

3. Strain then add your apple, and raspberries to a food processor or blender and process until smooth.

4. Strain, and serve.

About the Author

Jennifer Jones is an accomplished chef, devoted wife and loving mother of two who lives in Boulder, Colorado. As head chef at one of Colorado's most exclusive restaurants, Jennifer's culinary prowess has become legendary and she is often called over to the tables of the rich and famous to accept deep praise for her work.

The beautiful scenery of Boulder is often used as inspiration for some of Jennifer's artistically decorated dishes and the praise is just as much for her creative presentation as the exquisite taste of her food. Her use of greenery to bring out the delectable cuts of meat and fish that adorn the dinner plates is no less than a work of art, and she describes herself as an artist and not a chef.

Jones flourished under the mentorship of her professor at August Escoffier Culinary School of the Arts and went on to study at the Cordon Bleu to perfect her repertoire of international cuisine. While studying abroad, she kept close contact with her mentor from Escoffier, eventually marrying him when she came back to North America.

With all of that culinary ability, you would think some would rub off on the kids? Jennifer's two daughters are both excellent chefs in their own right and have plans to attend Escoffier like their parents. A culinary dynasty, perhaps?

Author's Afterthoughts

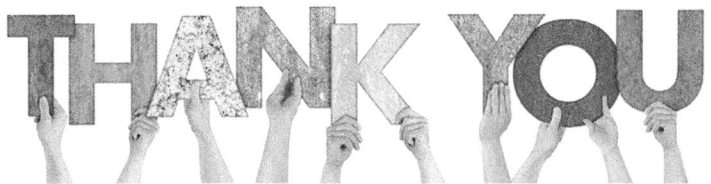

With so many books out there to choose from, I want to thank you for choosing this one and taking precious time out of your life to buy and read my work. Readers like you are the reason I take such passion in creating these books.

It is with gratitude and humility that I express how honored I am to become a part of your life and I hope that you take the same pleasure in reading this book as I did in writing it.

Can I ask one small favour? I ask that you write an honest and open review on Amazon of what you thought of the book. This will help other readers make an informed choice on whether to buy this book.

Sincerely,

Jennifer Jones

If you want to be the first to know about news, new books, events and giveaways, subscribe to my newsletter by clicking the link below

https://Jennifer-Jones.gr8.com

or Scan QR-code

Printed in Dunstable, United Kingdom